Complete Keto Beverages Cookbook

Delicious and Simple Beverages Recipes to Stay Fit for Women Over 50

Katie Attanasio

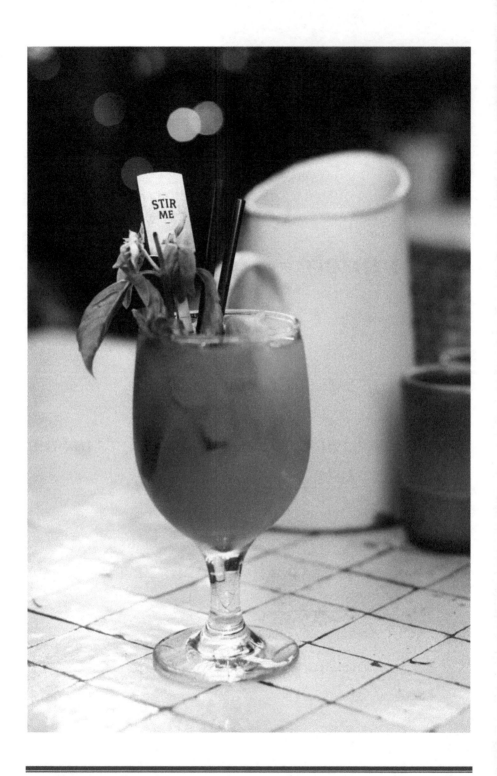

sources. Please consult a licensed professional before attempting any techniques outlined in this book.

By reading this document, the reader agrees that under no circumstances is the author responsible for any losses, direct or indirect, which are incurred as a result of the use of information contained within this document, including, but not limited to, — errors, omissions, or inaccuracies.

Table of Contents

Benefits of Keto for Women over 50

If you're a woman above 50 years of age, you may be keener on weight loss than you were at 30. Many women face a decreasing metabolism at this age at a rate of around 50 calories per day. It can be exceedingly difficult to regulate weight gain by slowing the metabolism combined with less exercise, muscle deterioration, and increased cravings.

To help lose some weight, there are several diet alternatives available, but the ketogenic diet has been one of the most common lately.

We have scientific advice here to give you the answers you are searching for if you would like to lose weight.

The advantages of Keto are numerous: from weight loss and improved energy levels to clinical uses. Keto is thought of more as a diet for weight loss. Low-carb keto diets, however, give women in their 50s some substantial additional benefits. A number of the advantages you may gain from a ketogenic diet are given below.

Reduced body fat

A lot of diets guarantee weight loss, but the weight seems to be mostly water in many cases. Keto improves the burning of fat and yields greater success than most other diets. Abdominal fat, properly called visceral fat, is also preferentially targeted by Keto.

In women over 50, abdominal fat appears to increase. This increases the risk of cardiac arrest and stroke. Abdominal fat development is primarily because of the hormonal shifts associated with menopause.

Increased insulin sensitivity

the carbohydrates get digested and convert into glucose. Your body releases the hormone insulin to ferry glucose into your liver and muscles when you eat carbohydrates. With age, though, the sensitivity of your body to insulin reduces, and that means that the glucose is more likely to be converted into and processed as fat, resulting in weight. With age, though, the sensitivity of your body to insulin reduces, and that means that the glucose is more likely to be converted into and processed as fat, resulting in weight loss.

Low carb diets improve insulin sensitivity. This means that it's not going to turn the few carbohydrates you consume into fat. Increased insulin sensitivity also helps to monitor blood glucose levels. Low blood glucose levels are inseparably related to better general health and a lower risk of type 2 diabetes.

Enhanced brain function

Things like mood swings, memory loss, and difficulty focusing are also encountered by menopausal women.

Anxiety and Depression can also cause them to suffer at times. This is because, during menopause, estrogen levels, the main female sex hormone, decrease, and that affects the glucose amount that enters your brain.

The keto diet gives an alternate source of fuel for your brain; ketones. Your brain works best on ketones, and on a low-carb diet, problems like mood swings and memory loss are far less likely.

The keto diet is also associated with a decreased risk of many neurological disorders, including Parkinson's disease and Alzheimer's disease, both of which are prominent in individuals over 50 years of age.

Reduced inflammation

The phase of aging can be rough on your body. In their 50s, menopausal women experience knee and hip pain and headaches, and other non-specific pain types.

Keto is a high-fat diet. Healthy anti-inflammatory fats that are expected to form part of the keto diet include:

Avocados and avocado oil Olive oil

Walnuts

Oily fish, such as salmon, sardines, and tuna.

Whereas foods like sugar, refined carbs, and processed foods are all linked to increased inflammation. So, these are not included in the keto diet.

Improved blood lipid profile

Many women face higher triglyceride levels and "bad" LDL cholesterol in their 50s. This may lead to a Heart Attack.

Low carb diets have been shown to reduce triglycerides and LDL cholesterol while being high in fat while increasing 'healthy' HDL cholesterol.

These improvements are associated with better cardiovascular health and a lower risk of cardiovascular disease.

Reduced blood pressure

The blood pressure of women appears to be lower than that of men. However, as you reach your 50s, that can change, and menopause begins to take hold.

A number of serious health conditions, including heart failure, kidney disease, and stroke, are related to high blood pressure. It has been shown that the keto diet improves reduce blood pressure levels.

Increased bone mass

Older women are vulnerable to bone loss, which can develop into osteoporosis if left untreated. This is a medical condition marked by thin, fracture-prone bones.

The nutrients that can interact with calcium absorption are replaced by Keto. Keto can help boost bone health and density, along with plenty of leafy green vegetables that are normally rich in calcium.

Less muscle loss

Females appear to lose muscle more rapidly in their 50s than women in their 20s, 30s, and 40s. The lack of muscle decreases your metabolic rate, leading to weight gain and making weight loss more difficult. Your strength would also be impaired by muscle loss, making daily tasks harder and more exhausting.

The ketogenic diet includes eating moderate quantities of protein, and for muscle perseverance, protein is essential. The protein comprises amino acids, and the basic components of muscle tissue are amino acids. It is easy to see that Keto can be very effective for weight loss and better health for women in their 50s. Going Keto means cutting out and substituting all of the things we know are unhealthy for foods that are rich in beneficial nutrients.

Keto, in short, is not just a diet for people who are overweight; it is a diet for anybody who wants a healthier and longer life!

Basic Benefits:

Weight Loss

A successful way to lose weight is by using a ketogenic diet. In reality, research indicates that a ketogenic diet can be as effective as a low-fat diet for weight loss. In essence, the ketogenic diet uses body fat as an energy source, so there are noticeable advantages to weight loss. The insulin levels drop significantly on Keto, which transforms the body into a machine for fat burning. It also resulted in declines in the amount of diastolic blood pressure and triglycerides.

A study of 34 older adults found that those who followed eight weeks of a ketogenic diet lost about five times as much overall body fat as those who adopted a low-fat diet.

Control Blood Sugar

You should consider a ketogenic diet if you are pre-diabetic or have Type 2 diabetes. A study of 349 individuals with type 2 diabetes showed that over two years, those who adopted a ketogenic diet lost an average of 11.9 kg. When considering the relation between weight and type 2 diabetes, this is a significant advantage. They also experienced better blood sugar control, and during the study, the use of some blood sugar medicines among participants decreased.

Mental Focus

For improved mental performance, many individuals use the ketogenic diet specifically.

The keto diet can help reduce and delay the progression of Alzheimer's disease symptoms. Although further research is needed, one study showed that the diet improved Parkinson's disease symptoms. Some research indicates that traumatic brain injuries may boost the effects of the diet.

Increased Energy & Normalized Hunger

You can feel more motivated throughout the day by offering your body a healthier and more stable energy form. It is proven that fats are the most efficient molecule to be burned as fuel.

Epilepsy

The ketogenic diet has been used to effectively treat epilepsy since the 1900s. Research has shown that in epileptic children, a ketogenic diet can cause a substantial reduction in seizures. For children who have untreated epilepsy today, it is also one of the most widely utilized treatments. One of the key advantages of the ketogenic diet for epilepsy is that it enables fewer medicines while also having excellent control.

Studies have also demonstrated substantial results in adults treated with Keto in the last couple of years.

Cholesterol & Blood Pressure

The reduction of triglyceride levels and cholesterol levels connected with arterial accumulation has been improved through a keto diet. More precisely, low-carb high-fat diets display a dramatic rise in HDL and a drop in LDL particle concentration. The research on ketogenic diets also shows greater improvement over other diets in blood pressure.

Insulin Resistance

When left uncontrolled, insulin resistance can escalate to type II diabetes. A significant amount of research indicates that a ketogenic diet helps individuals reduce their insulin levels to safe ranges.

Even if you're athletic, by eating foods rich in omega-3 fatty acids, you will gain from insulin regulation on Keto.

Acne

When you turn to a keto diet, it's normal to report changes in your skin.

Here's one study showing reductions in lesions and inflammation of the skin while transitioning to a low-carb diet.

Another study shows that high carb eating and intensified acne are likely related, so Keto may likely help.

Polycystic ovary syndrome

A ketogenic diet helps reduce the level of insulin, which is mostly responsible for this disease.

Women's Hormones And The Keto Diet

Dr. Natasha Turner, ND, states that several of her female patients would initially lose weight. They then plateau and start gaining back all the weight and extra too. Obviously, this is not the perfect case. Cutting carbs suddenly can bring stress to the bodies of women.

At first, an increase in the stress hormone (cortisol) may be caused. Belly fat, Insulin resistance, and diabetes are associated with cortisol. The reduction of protein consumption in favor of more fats on the keto diet is one reason for this rise. Dr. Turner says that about 46 g of carbs a day are required for women (more for active women).

But that does not always qualify for the keto diet. This means the body will start eating for stores in muscles for food. Muscle wasting induces stress and cortisol spikes. Uh, not good.

Increased cortisol can alter the ratio of sex hormones in females over time. More testosterone, estrogen, and less progesterone start to be formed by the body. This could lead to disorders that are reproductive and hormonal. The exact reversal of the principle behind the diet.

The third hormonal problem has to do with the production of estrogen as well. Increased dietary fat is associated with increased development of estrogen in women. The higher the amount of estrogen, the more the thyroid is inhibited, according to Dr. Turner.

Since a healthy metabolism (weight management, sex drive cognition, and mood) is important to the thyroid, suppressing it is not pleasant. It can potentially lead to weight gain.

50 Essential Beverages Recipes

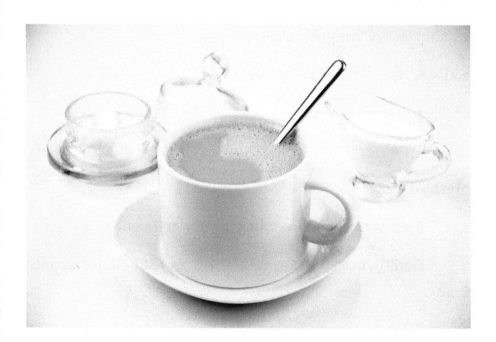

1   Coffee With Cream

Servings: 1 | **Time:** 5 mins | **Difficulty:** Easy

ents per serving: Calories: 203 kcal | Fat: 21g | Carbohydrates: 2g | Protein: 2g | Fiber: 0g

Ingredients

1/4 Cup Heavy Whipping Cream

2 Tbsps. Nuts, Crushed (Optional)

3/4 Cup Brewed Coffee

Method

1.   Brew your coffee according to your preference.

2.   Slightly heat the cream in a pan and stir till it becomes frothy.

3.   Take a cup and mix the warm cream and coffee in it.

4.   Serve hot with crushed nuts on top or as it is.

2   Keto Coffee

Servings: 2 | **Time:** 5 mins | **Difficulty**: Easy

Nutrients per serving: Calories: 260 kcal | Fat: 27.7g | Carbohydrates: 1.05g | Protein: 1.08g | Fiber: 0g

Ingredients

2   Tbsps. Coconut Oil Or MCT Oil

2 Tbsps. Butter, Unsalted (Grass-Fed)

2 Cups Brewed Coffee

1 Tsp. Vanilla Extract (Optional)

1 Tbsp. Heavy Whipping Cream (Optional)

Method

1.   Brew your coffee according to your preference.

2.   Blend the coffee with unsalted butter, coconut or MCT oil, vanilla extract, and whipping cream if you want, in a blender for about a minute or until it becomes frothy.

3.   Pour out the keto coffee in your favorite mugs and enjoy.

3   Vegan Keto Golden Milk

Servings: 1 | **Time:** 5 mins | **Difficulty**: Easy

Nutrients per serving: Calories: 303 kcal | Fat: 31.1g | Carbohydrates: 2.7g | Protein: 2.1g | Fiber: 2g

Ingredients

2 Tsps. Ginger, Fresh & Peeled

2 Tbsps. MCT Oil

1 & 1/2 Cup Almond Milk, Unsweetened

2 Tsps. Erythritol

1/4 Tsp. Cinnamon, Ground

2 Ice Cubes

3/4 Tsp. Turmeric Powder

1/4 Tsp. Vanilla Extract

Sea Salt, To Taste

Method

1. Combine all the ingredients in a blender and mix for about a quarter or half a minute.

2. For the strong taste of turmeric and ginger, blend longer.

3. Decant into the glass or mug and sprinkle powdered cinnamon on top before serving.

4   Keto Creamy Chocolate Smoothie

Servings: 2 | **Time:** 10 mins | **Difficulty:** Easy

Nutrients per serving: Calories: 593.3 kcal | Fat: 55.7g | Carbohydrates: 7.7g | Protein: 10.6g | Fiber: 11.7g

Ingredients

1 Tbsp. Almond Butter

1 Tsp. Coconut Oil

1/2 Avocado

1 Tbsp. Flax Meal

1 & 1/4 Cups Almond Milk, Unsweetened

1 Tbsp. Cocoa Powder, Unsweetened

1/4 Cup Heavy Whipping Cream

Liquid Stevia, To Taste

Method

1.   Combine all the ingredients in a blender and mix until a smooth consistency is attained.

2.   Decant into the serving glass and top with cocoa powdered and whipped cream if you want.

5   Keto Pumpkin Pie Spice Latte

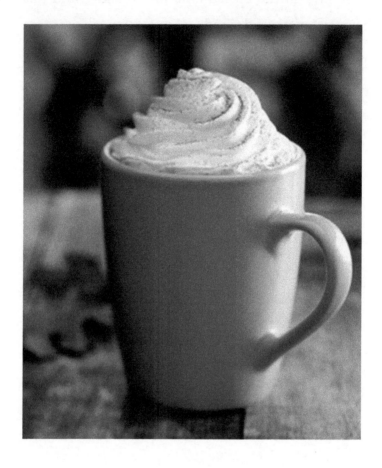

Servings: 3 | **Time**: 10 mins | **Difficulty**: Easy

Nutrients per serving: Calories: 136.28 kcal | Fat: 19.83g | Carbohydrates: 2.49g | Protein: 0.68g | Fiber: 1.79g

Ingredients

2 Tbsps. Butter

1/2 Tsp. Cinnamon, Powdered

1 Cup Coconut Milk

2 Cups Brewed Coffee

2 Tsps. Pumpkin Pie Spice

1/4 Cup Pumpkin Puree

1 Tsp. Vanilla Extract

2 Tbsps. Heavy Whipping Cream

15 Drops Liquid Stevia

Method

1.   Pour the coconut milk, butter, pumpkin puree, and spices into a small saucepan and heat over a medium-low flame.

2.   Once the mixture starts to bubble, add the coffee, and mix well.

3.   Remove from the heat and add the whipped cream and liquid Stevia. Mix well to blend the contents until frothy.

4.   Decant in the serving mug and a dollop of whipped cream on top.

6   Blueberry Banana Bread Smoothie

Servings: 2 | **Time:** 10 mins | **Difficulty:** Easy

Nutrients per serving: Calories: 270 kcal | Fat: 23.31g | Carbohydrates: 4.66g | Protein: 3.13g | Fiber: 5.65g

Ingredients

1/4 Cup Blueberries

2 Tbsps. MCT Oil

2 1 & 1/2 Tsps. Banana Extract

Cups Vanilla Coconut Milk, Unsweetened

1 Tbsp. Chia Seeds

3 Tbsps. Golden Flaxseed Meal

10 Drop Liquid Stevia

1/4 Tsp. Xanthan Gum

Method

1.   Combine all the ingredients in a blender and let it sit for a few minutes to allow the chia and flax seeds to soak some moisture.

2.   Then blend for a minute or two until a smooth consistency is attained.

3.   Serve in the glasses and enjoy.

7   Blackberry Chocolate Shake

Servings: 2 | **Time:** 5 mins | **Difficulty:** Easy

Nutrients per serving: Calories: 346 kcal | Fat: 34.17g | Carbohydrates: 4.8g | Protein: 2.62g | Fiber: 7.4g

Ingredients

1/4 Cup Blackberries

2 Tbsps. MCT Oil

1 Cup Coconut Milk, Unsweetened

1/4 Tsp. Xanthan Gum

2 Tbsps. Cocoa Powder

12 Drops Liquid Stevia

7 Ice Cubes

Method

1.   Combine all the ingredients in a blender and blend for a minute or two until a smooth consistency is attained.

2.   Serve in the glasses and enjoy.

8   Dairy-Free Dark Chocolate Shake

Servings: 2 | **Time:** 5 mins | **Difficulty:** Easy

Nutrients per serving: Calories: 349.35 kcal | Fat: 33.15g | Carbohydrates: 5.73g | Protein: 7.2g | Fiber: 6.1g

Ingredients

1/2 Avocado

1/2 Cup Coconut Cream, Chilled

2 Tbsps. Hulled Hemp Seeds

2 Tbsps. Dark Chocolate (Low Carb)

1/2 Cup Almond Milk

1 Tbsp. Cocoa Powder

2 Tbsps. Powdered Erythritol, To Taste

Flake Salt, To Taste

1 Cup Ice

Method

1.   Put the cocoa powder, hemp seeds, erythritol, and dark chocolate in a blender and mix until the chocolate is chopped.

2.   Add the remaining ingredients and blend for a minute or two until a smooth consistency is attained.

3.   Pour in the serving glasses and enjoy.

9   Keto Meal Replacement Shake

Servings: 2 | **Time**: 5 mins | **Difficulty:** Easy

Nutrients per serving: Calories: 453 kcal | Fat: 42.6g | Carbohydrates: 6.9g | Protein: 8.8g | Fiber: 8.1g

Ingredients

1/2 Avocado

2 Tbsps. Almond Butter

1 Cup Almond Or Coconut Milk, Unsweetened

1/4 Tsp. Vanilla Extract

1/2 Tsp. Cinnamon, Powdered

2 Tbsps. Golden Flaxseed Meal

1/8 Tsp. Salt

2 Tbsp. Cocoa Powder

1/2 Cup Heavy Cream

15 Drops Liquid Stevia

8 Ice Cubes

Method

1.   Combine all the ingredients in a blender and blend for a minute or two until a smooth consistency is attained.

2.   Serve in the glasses and enjoy.

10   Keto Iced Coffee

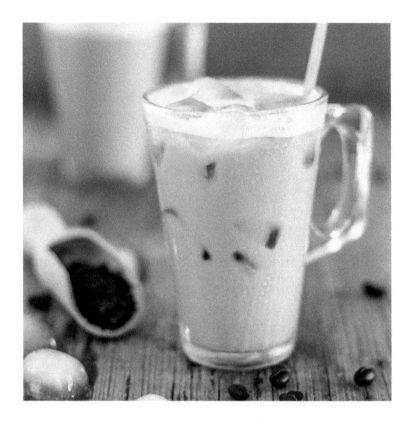

Servings: 1 | **Time**: 5 mins | **Difficulty**: Easy

Nutrients per serving: Calories: 160 kcal | Fat: 16.1g | Carbohydrates: 1.5g | Protein: 1.6g | Fiber: 0g

dients

3 Tbsps. Heavy Cream

5 Drops Liquid Stevia

1 Cup Brewed Coffee

1/2 Tsp. Vanilla Extract (Optional)

Ice Cubes, To Taste

Method

1.   Brew your coffee according to your preference and let it cool down to room temperature.

2.   Combine the coffee with all the other ingredients in a blender and blend for about a minute or until it becomes frothy.

3.   Pour the iced coffee in your favorite mug and enjoy.

11   Low-Carb Ginger Smoothie

Servings: 2 | **Time:** 5 mins | **Difficulty:** Easy

Nutrients per serving: Calories: 83 kcal | Fat: 8g | Carbohydrates: 3g | Protein: 1g | Fiber: 1g

Ingredients

2 Tbsps. Spinach, Frozen

1/3 Cup Coconut Milk Or Cream, Unsweetened

2 Tsps. Ginger, Fresh & Grated

2 Tbsps. Lime Juice, Divided

2/3 Cup Water

For Garnishing:

1/2 Tsp. Fresh Ginger, Grated

Method

1.   Combine all the ingredients in a blender and adjust the lime juice amount as per your taste.

2.   Blend the mixture for a minute or until a smooth consistency is attained.

3.   Serve with grated ginger on top.

12 Whipped Dairy-Free Low-Carb Dalgona Coffee

Servings: 2 | **Time:** 5 mins | **Difficulty:** Easy

Nutrients per serving: Calories: 40 kcal | Fat: 2g | Carbohydrates: 1g | Protein: 1g | Fiber: 1g

Ingredients

2 Tbsps. Water, Hot

1 & 1/2 Cups Coconut Or Almond Milk, Unsweetened

1 & 1/2 Tbsps. Erythritol

1 & 1/2 Tbsps. Espresso Instant Coffee Powder

1/2 Cup Ice Cubes

1 Tsp. Vanilla Extract (Optional)

Method

1.   Take a narrow glass and combine the coffee powder, hot water, and erythritol in it and blend them well with an

immersion blender for about 3 minutes or till the mixture becomes creamy and light in color.

2.   Take two glasses, fill two-third of them with ice and then pour the almond or coconut milk in it along with vanilla extract if you want. Mix them well.

3.   Put the spoonful of the creamy coffee mixture on the top of each glass and stir before serving.

13   Keto Eggnog

Servings: 4 | **Time:** 10 mins | **Difficulty:** Easy

Nutrients per serving: Calories: 249 kcal | Fat: 24g | Carbohydrates: 6g | Protein: 3g | Fiber: 1g

Ingredients

1/4 Cup Orange Juice

2 Egg Yolks

1/2 Tbsp. Orange Zest

1/4 Tbsp. Vanilla

1/2 Tsp. Erythritol, Powdered

1/8 Tsp. Nutmeg, Ground

1 Cup Heavy Whipping Cream

4 Tbsps. Bourbon Or Brandy (Optional)

Method

1.   Combine egg yolks, vanilla extract, and erythritol in a deep bowl and whisk the mixture well until it becomes fluffy.

2.   Add in the orange juice, orange zest, and whipping cream. Mix well until a smooth consistency is attained.

3.   Pour the eggnog n the serving glasses and refrigerate for about 15 minutes.

4.   Finally, serve with a sprinkle of nutmeg on top.

14   Iced Tea

Servings: 2 | **Time:** 2 hrs. & 10 mins | **Difficulty**: Easy

Nutrients per serving: Calories: 0 kcal | Fat: 0g | Carbohydrates: 0g | Protein: 0g | Fiber: 0g

Ingredients

1 Tea Bag

2 Cups Cold Water

1 Cup Ice Cubes

1/3 Cup Sliced Lemon or Fresh Mint Leaves

Method

1.   Put the teabag and lemon slices or mint leaves in a cup of cold water in a pitcher and put in the refrigerator for an hour or two.

2.   Take the tea bag, and lemon slices or mint leaves out of the water. Substitute them with new ones if you want.

3.   Pour in another cup of water and ice cubes in the pitcher and serve.

15   Flavored Water

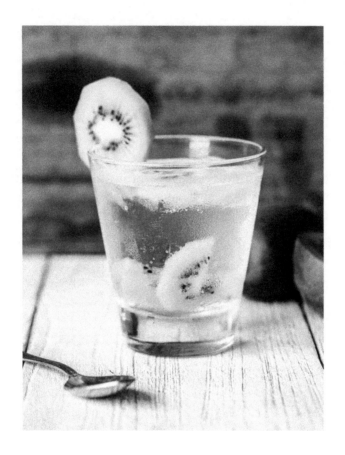

Servings: 4 | **Time:** 5 mins | **Difficulty:** Easy

Nutrients per serving: Calories: 0 kcal | Fat: 0g | Carbohydrates: 0g | Protein: 0g | Fiber: 0g

Ingredients

2 Cups Ice Cubes

Flavoring, e.g., Fresh Mint Or Raspberries, Or Sliced Cucumber
4 Cups Cold Water

Method

1.   Take a pitcher and add cold water along with flavorings in
it.

2.   Refrigerate it for about 30 minutes and then serve.

16   Butter Coffee

Servings: 1 | **Time:** 5 mins | **Difficulty**: Easy

Nutrients per serving: Calories: 0 kcal | Fat: 37g | Carbohydrates: 0g | Protein: 1g | Fiber: 0g

Ingredients

2 Tbsps. Butter, Unsalted

1 Tbsp. Coconut Or MCT Oil

1 Cup Freshly Brewed Coffee, Hot

Method

1.   Brew your coffee according to your preference, and let it cool down a bit.

2.   Combine the coffee with all the other ingredients in a blender and blend for about a minute or until it becomes frothy.

3.   Pour the butter coffee in your favorite mug and enjoy.

17 Keto Hot Chocolate

Servings: 1 | **Time:** 5 mins | **Difficulty:** Easy

Nutrients per serving: Calories: 216 kcal | Fat: 23g | Carbohydrates: 1g | Protein: 1g | Fiber: 2g

Ingredients

1 Cup Boiling Water

2 & 1/2 Tsps. Powdered Erythritol

2 Tbsps. Butter, Unsalted

1/4 Tsp. Vanilla Extract

1 Tbsp. Cocoa Powder

Method

1.   Combine all the ingredients in a full-sized mug and blend well with an immersion blender until it becomes frothy.

2.   Serve hot and enjoy.

18 Dairy-Free Keto Latte

Servings: 2 | **Time:** 5 mins | **Difficulty:** Easy

Nutrients per serving: Calories: 191 kcal | Fat: 18g | Carbohydrates: 1g | Protein: 6g | Fiber: 0g

Ingredients

1 & 1/2 Cups Boiling Water

2 Tbsps. Coconut Oil

1 Tsp. Ground Ginger Or Pumpkin Pie Spice

2 Eggs

1/8 Tsp. Vanilla Extract

Method

1.   Combine all the ingredients in a blender and blend for a few seconds.

2.   Do not let the eggs cook in the boiling water and serve instantly.

19 Low-Carb Vegan Vanilla Protein Shake

Servings: 1 | **Time:** 10 mins | **Difficulty:** Easy

Nutrients per serving: Calories: 449 kcal | Fat: 34g | Carbohydrates: 8g | Protein: 28g | Fiber: 4g

Ingredients

4 Tbsps. Pea Protein Powder, Unflavored

1/2 Cup Almond Milk, Unsweetened

2 Tbsps. Cauliflower Rice, Frozen

1 Tbsp. Almond Butter

1/2 Cup Coconut Milk

1 Tsp. Vanilla Extract

1/2 Tsp. Cinnamon, Ground

Method

1.   Combine all the ingredients in a blender and blend the mixture for a minute or until a smooth consistency is attained.

2.   Decant in a serving glass and enjoy.

20 Electrolyte Elixir

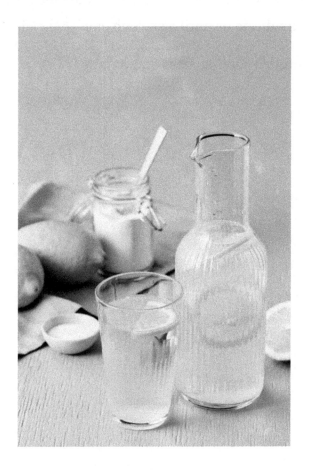

Servings: 4 | **Time**: 1 min | **Difficulty:** Easy

Nutrients per serving: Calories: 7 kcal | Fat: 0.1g | Carbohydrates: 2g | Protein: 0.1g | Fiber: 0g

Ingredients

1/2 Cup Lemon Juice, Fresh

1/2 Tsp. Magnesium

1 Tsp. Salt

8 Cups Water

Method

1. Combine all the ingredients in a pitcher and stir well.

2. Decant in serving glasses and enjoy.

21   Keto Chai Latte

Servings: 2 | **Time:** 5 mins | **Difficulty:** Beginner

Nutrients per serving: Calories: 133 kcal | Fat: 14g | Carbohydrates: 1g | Protein: 1g | Fiber: 0g

Ingredients

2 Cups Boiling Water

1/3 Cup Heavy Whipping Cream

1 Tbsp. Chai Tea

Method

1.   According to the package instructions, brew the tea in boiling water.

2.   In a saucepan or microwave, heat the cream and pour it into the tea and serve.

22 Sugar-Free Mulled Wine

Servings: 8 | **Time:** 15 mins | **Difficulty:** Beginner

Nutrients per serving: Calories: 82 kcal | Fat: 0.1g | Carbohydrates: 3g | Protein: 0.1g | Fiber: 0g

Ingredients

2 Cinnamon Sticks

1 & 1/2 Tsps. Orange Zest, Dried

1 Star Anise

2 Tsps. Ginger, Dried

1 Tsp. Green Cardamom Seeds

3 Cups White Or Red Wine, With Or Without Alcohol

1 Tsp. Cloves

1 Tbsp. Vanilla Extract (Optional)

Method

1.   Combine all the ingredients in a saucepan and simmer over medium-low flame for about 5-10 minutes. Do not bring to boil.

2.   Remove from the heat and let the mixture sit overnight for a strong taste of spices.

3.   Strain the wine and serve hot with snacks or nuts.

23 Co-Keto (Puerto Rican Coconut Eggnog)

Servings: 2 | **Time:** 5 mins | **Difficulty:** Easy

Nutrients per serving: Calories: 563kcal | Fat: 56g| Carbohydrates: 7g | Protein: 7g| Fiber: 0g

Ingredients

3 & 1/3 Cups Coconut Cream

2 Cups Heavy Whipping Cream

4 Egg Yolks, Beaten

1 & 2/3 Cups Coconut Milk, Unsweetened

1 Cup Rum

1/2 Cup Warm Water

2 Tbsps. Coconut Oil

1 Tbsp. Vanilla Extract Stevia, To Taste

2 Tsps. Cinnamon, Ground

1/4 Tsp. Ginger, Ground

1/4 Tsp. Nutmeg, Ground

1/4 Tsp. Cloves, Ground

Method

1.   Heat the beaten egg yolks and whipping cream together in a double boiler, constantly stirring until a smooth consistency is attained and the temperature reaches 160°F.

2.   Add the coconut oil and mix well until thick and smooth.

3.   Pour this mixture into a blender and add all the other ingredients. Blend well and then transfer to the glass bottles and let chill.

24 Cinnamon Coffee

Servings: 1 | **Time:** 5 mins | **Difficulty:** Easy

Nutrients per serving: Calories: 660 kcal | Fat: 60g | Carbohydrates: 7g | Protein: 13g | Fiber: 7g

Ingredients

1/2 Tsp. Brown Sugar

1/8 Tsp. Cinnamon, Powdered Whipped Cream (Optional)

1 Cup Coffee

Method

1.   According to the package instructions, brew the coffee.

2.   Add the brown sugar and cinnamon powder to it and stir well.

3.   Put a dollop of whipped cream on top if you want.

25 Sugar-Free Caramel Brulee Latte

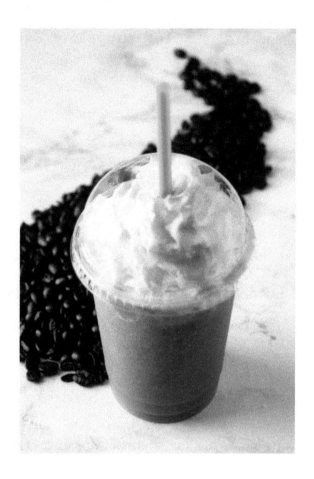

Servings: 2 | **Time:** 2 mins | **Difficulty**: Easy

Nutrients per serving: Calories: 106 kcal | Fat: 11g | Carbohydrates: 1g | Protein: 1g |

Ingredients

2 Tbsps. Caramel Syrup

2 Cups Brewed Coffee

4 Tbsps. Coconut Milk Or Heavy Whipped Cream

Method

1.   Brew your coffee according to your preference and add one Tbsp. of caramel syrup and 2 Tbsps. of coconut milk or heavy cream in each cup.

2.   Top with a dollop of whipped cream or caramel if you want and serve.

26 Pumpkin Spice Latte Milkshakes

Servings: 3 | **Time:** 15 mins | **Difficulty**: Easy

Nutrients per serving (with 2 Tbsps. whipped coconut cream per shake): Calories: 364 kcal | Fat: 18.52g| Carbohydrates: 5.48g | Protein: 2.3g| Fiber: 1.83g

Ingredients

1 Cup Keto Vanilla Ice Cream

1/3 Cup Almond Milk

1/3 Cup Water

2 Tbsps. Pumpkin Puree

1 & 1/2 Tsp. Instant Coffee

1 Tsp. Pumpkin Pie Spice

Coconut Whipped Cream:

2 Tbsps. Sugar (Low Carb)

1 & 3/4 Cups Coconut Milk

Method

1.   Put the coconut milk in the refrigerator overnight, take the thick cream off the milk top, and put it in a bowl. Save the milk for other recipes.

2.   Whisk in the low carb sugar in the coconut cream until your desired consistency is attained.

3.   Combine all the other ingredients in a blender and blend for a few minutes until it becomes smooth.

4.   Decant in your preferred glasses and top with coconut whipped cream.

27　Keto Russian Coffee

Servings: 2 | **Time:** 2 mins | **Difficulty:** Easy

Nutrients per serving: Calories: 214 kcal | Fat: 22g | Carbohydrates: 3g | Protein: 2g | Fiber: 1g

Ingredients

1/3 Cup Vanilla Vodka

4 Tbsps. Almond Milk, Unsweetened

2 Tbsps. Stevia

2 Cups Brewed Coffee Milk Foam (Optional)

1/4 Cup Heavy Cream

2 Tbsps. French Vanilla Whipped Foam Topping (Sugar-Free)

1 Stick Of Cinnamon

1/4 Tsp. Vanilla Extract

Method

1.   Brew coffee according to your preference and divide it into two cups. Stir in half of the almond milk, Stevia, and vodka in each cup.

2.   Put the milk foam on top if you want.

3.   To make milk foam, combine all its ingredients in a jar and mix well until the mixture becomes frothy. Microwave for 10 sec and then put a dollop on each serving.

28   Creamy Matcha Latte

Servings: 1 | **Time:** 6 mins | **Difficulty:** Easy

Nutrients per serving: Calories: 255 kcal | Fat: 22.8g| Carbohydrates: 5.3g | Protein: 2.33g | Fiber: 1.3g

Ingredients

1/8 Tsp. Pink Sea Salt

1/3 Cup Almond Milk, Unsweetened

1 Tsp. Matcha Tea

2/3 Cup Coconut Milk Stevia, To Taste

4 Drops Vanilla Extract (Optional)

Method

1.   Take a saucepan and add both kinds of milk to it. Heat until it starts to bubble and add the remaining ingredients to it.

2.   Mix well and serve in separate cups.

29   Keto Avocado Smoothie

Servings: 2 | **Time:** 10 mins | **Difficulty:** Easy

Nutrients per serving: Calories: 232 kcal | Fat: 22.4g | Carbohydrates: 6.9g | Protein: 1.7g | Fiber: 2.8g

Ingredients

1/2 Tsp. Turmeric Powder

1 Tsp. Fresh Ginger, Grated

1/4 Cup Almond Milk

3/4 Cup Coconut Milk

1/2 Avocado

1 Tsp. Lime Or Lemon Juice

1 Cup Ice, Crushed

Stevia, To Taste

Method

1. Combine all the ingredients in a blender and blend until a smooth consistency is attained.

2. Pour in your favorite glasses and enjoy.

30 Avocado Mint Green Keto Smoothie

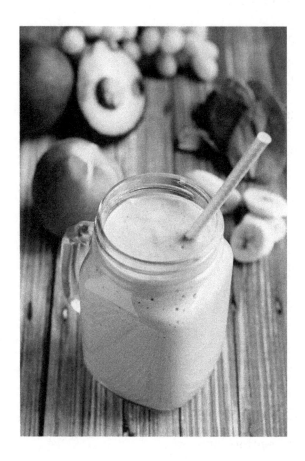

Servings: 1 | **Time:** 2 mins | **Difficulty:** Easy

Nutrients per serving: Calories: 223 kcal | Fat: 23g | Carbohydrates: 5g | Protein: 1g | Fiber: 1g

nts

1/2 Cup Almond Milk

5-6 Mint Leaves

1/2 Avocado

3/4 Cup Coconut Milk

1/2 Tsp. Lime Juice

1 & 1/2 Cups Ice,

Crushed Stevia, To Taste

3 Cilantro Sprigs

1/4 Tsp. Vanilla Extract

Method

1.   Combine all the ingredients in a blender, except ice, and blend until it becomes smooth.

2.   Then, add the crushed ice and blend again till the desired consistency.

3.   Pour into glasses and serve.

31   Keto Skinny Margaritas

Servings: 2 | **Time**: 10 mins | **Difficulty**: Easy

Nutrients per serving: Calories: 102 kcal | Fat: 1g | Carbohydrates: 1g | Protein: 1g

Ingredients

1/3 Cup Tequila

1 Tbsp. Warm Water

2 Tbsps. Lime Juice

Ice Cubes, To Taste

Stevia, To Taste

Coarse Salt, For Glass's Rim

Method

1.   Mix the warm water and Stevia in a bowl and put squeeze the lime juice in another bowl.

2.   Take a jar and combine the lime juice, sweetener syrup, and the tequila in it. Close the lid of the jar and shake it well to mix the contents.

3.   Slightly wet the rim of two cocktail glasses and line with salt, and pour the margarita in them.

4.   Add the ice in them and garnish with a slice of fresh lime if you want.

32 Iced Keto Matcha Green Tea Latte

Servings: 1 | **Time:** 1 min | **Difficulty:** Easy

Nutrients per serving: Calories: 36 kcal | Fat: 2.5g | Carbohydrates: 0.8g | Protein: 1.6g | Fiber: 0.8g

Ingredients

5 Drops Vanilla Stevia

1 Tsp. Matcha Powder

1 Cup Coconut Or Vanilla Almond Milk, Unsweetened

Ice, To Taste

Method

1.   Combine all ingredients in a blender and blend for a few minutes until a smooth consistency is attained and match if completely dissolved.

2.   Add ice in your preferred quantity and enjoy.

33 Spiced Gingerbread Coffee

Servings: 1 | **Time:** 2 mins | **Difficulty**: Easy

Nutrients per serving: Calories: 108 kcal | Fat: 11.2g | Carbohydrates: 1.5g | Protein: 1g

Ingredients

1 Cup Hot Brewed Coffee

1 Tbsp. Heavy Cream

1/2 Tsp. Sukrin Gold

1 & 1/2 Tsps. Sukrin Gold Fiber Syrup

1/4 Tsp. Ginger, Ground

1/8 Tsp. Cloves, Ground

1/8 Tsp. Cinnamon, Ground

Whipped Cream

Method

1.   Combine all the ingredients in a mug except cloves and cream. Mix well until the spices are blended thoroughly.

2.   Add a dollop of whipped cream on top and sprinkle the ground cloves on it.

nut Milk Strawberry Smoothie

Servings: 2 | **Time:** 2 mins | **Difficulty:** Easy

Nutrients per serving: Calories: 397 kcal | Fat: 37g | Carbohydrates: 15g | Protein: 6g | Fiber: 5g

Ingredients

2 Tbsps. Almond Butter, Smooth

1 Cup Coconut Milk, Unsweetened

3/4 Tsp. Stevia (Optional)

1 Cup Strawberries, Frozen

Method

1.   Combine all the ingredients in a blender and mix until a smooth consistency is attained.

2.   Decant into the serving glasses and enjoy.

35 Peanut Butter Chocolate Keto Milkshake

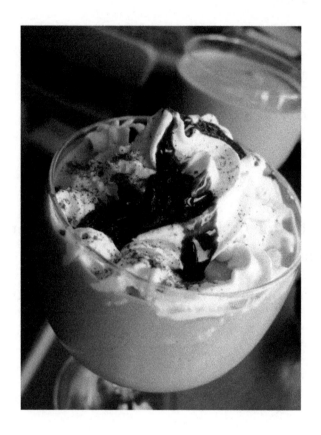

Servings: 1 | **Time:** 1 min | **Difficulty**: Easy

Nutrients per serving: Calories: 79 kcal | Fat: 5.7g | Carbohydrates: 6.4g | Protein: 3.6g | Fiber: 3.3g

Ingredients

5 Drops Stevia

1/8 Tsp. Sea Salt

1 Tbsp. Peanut Butter Powder, Unsweetened

1 Cup Coconut Milk, Unsweetened

1 Tbsp. Cocoa Powder, Unsweetened

Method

1.   Combine all the ingredients in a blender and mix until a smooth consistency is attained.

2.   Decant into the serving glasses and enjoy.

36 Sugar-Free Fresh Squee Lemonade

Servings: 8 | **Time:** 10 mins | **Difficulty:** Easy

Nutrients per serving: Calories: 5 kcal | Fat: 1g | Carbohydrates: 2g | Protein: 1g | Fiber: 1g

Ingredients

8 Cups Water

1 Tsp. Lemon Monkfruit Drops

4 Slices Lemon (Optional)

3/4 Cup Lemon Juice

Ice (Optional)

Method

1.   Combine all the ingredients in a pitcher and stir well to mix.

2.   Chill in the refrigerator or add ice to it before serving.

3.   Put the lemon slices in it if you want.

37   Cucumber Mint Water

Servings: 16 | **Time:** 5 mins | **Difficulty**: Easy

Nutrients per serving: Calories: 3 kcal | Fat: 0g | Carbohydrates: 0g | Protein: 0g | Fiber: 0g

Ingredients

8 Cups Water

3/4 Cup Cucumber Slices

1 Tbsps. Mint Leaves

Method

1.   Press the mint leaves in a pitcher with the help of a spoon and add the other ingredients to it.

2.   Chill it in the refrigerator for an hour and then enjoy.

38 Caramel Apple Drink

Servings: 1 | **Time:** 10 mins | **Difficulty**: Easy

Nutrients per serving: Calories: 76 kcal | Fat: 3g | Carbohydrates: 16g | Protein: 1g | Fiber: 14g

Ingredients

2 Cups Water

1 Tbsp. Caramel Syrup

1 Tbsp. Apple Cider Vinegar (Raw)

1/8 Tsp. Allspice

1/8 Tsp. Nutmeg, Ground

1/8 Tsp. Orange Zest, Dried

1 Cinnamon Stick, Halved

3 Whole Cloves

1/4 Cup Vanilla Whipped Cream (Optional)

1/8 Tsp. Cinnamon, Ground (Optional)

5 Drops Stevia (Optional)

Method

1.   Take the water in a pan and put the allspice, cinnamon stick halves, and cloves in it. Boil the water and then let it sit for 2-3 minutes off the heat, with the lid on.

2.   Strain the spice water into a large mug and put the caramel syrup and apple cider vinegar in it. Stir well and add Stevia or ground cinnamon if you want.

3.   Put a dollop of whipped cream on top if you ant and drizzle some caramel syrup if you want.

39   Keto Frosty Chocolate Shake

Servings: 1 | **Time:** 10 mins | **Difficulty:** Easy

Nutrients per serving: Calories: 346 kcal | Fat: 36g | Carbohydrates: 8.4g | Protein: 4g | Fiber: 4g

Ingredients

5 Tbsps. Almond Milk, Unsweetened

2 Tbsps. Cocoa Powder

1 & 1/2 Tsps. Truvia

1/8 Tsp. Vanilla Extract (Sugar-Free)

6 Tbsps. Heavy Whipping Cream

Method

1.   Combine all the ingredients and whisk well to make a fluffy peak of cream.

2.   Freeze the mixture for 20 minutes and then crack it open with a fork.

3.   Chill it as per your preference and serve cold.

40 Strawberry Avocado Smoothie

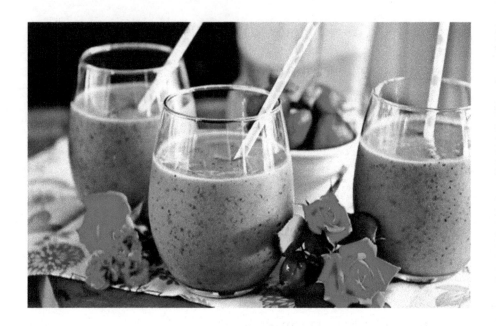

Servings: 2 | **Time:** 2 mins | **Difficulty:** Easy

Nutrients per serving: Calories: 165 kcal | Fat: 14g| Carbohydrates: 11g | Protein: 2g | Fiber: 7g

Ingredients

1 & 1/2 Cups Coconut Milk

1 Tsp. Stevia

1 Avocado

1 Tbsp. Lime Juice

2/3 Cup Strawberries, Frozen

1/2 Cup Ice

Method

1.   Combine all the ingredients in a blender and blend until a smooth consistency is attained.

2.   Pour in your favorite glasses and enjoy.

41 Almond Berry Mini Cheesecake Smoothies

Servings: 2 | **Time:** 10 mins | **Difficulty**: Easy

Nutrients per serving: Calories: 165 kcal | Fat: 8.6g | Carbohydrates: 16.8g | Protein: 7g | Fiber: 4.4g

Ingredients

1 Cup Almond Or Coconut Milk, Chilled

2 Tbsps. Almond Or Coconut Flour

2 Cups Mixed Berries, Frozen

1 Tbsp. Almond Butter, Smooth

1/2 Cup Cottage Cheese, Organic

1 Tsp. Nuts Or Almonds, Toasted & Crushed

1 Tsp. Vanilla Extract

1/8 Tsp. Cinnamon

Stevia, To Taste (Optional)

Method

1.   Combine all the ingredients in a blender, except crushed nuts, and blend until a smooth consistency is attained.

2.   You can add Stevia if you want and pour it into cups.

3.   Top with crushed and toasted nuts and serve.

42   Hemp Milk And Nut Milk

Servings: 4 | **Time:** 12 hrs. 15 mins | **Difficulty**: Easy

Nutrients per serving: Calories: 44 kcal | Fat: 3.6g | Carbohydrates: 1.7g | Protein: 1.5g | Fiber: 0.9g

Ingredients

Nut milk:

4 Cups Water

1/8 Tsp. Sea Salt

1 Cup Raw Nuts (Pecan, Almond, Walnut, Cashew, etc.)

1 Tsp. Vanilla Extract (Optional)

1/3 Cup Maple Syrup (Optional)

For Hemp Milk:

3 Cups Water

1/8 Tsp. Sea Salt

1/2 Cup Hulled Hemp Seed

1/4 Cup Maple Syrup (Optional)

1 Tsp. Vanilla Extract (Optional)

Method

Nut Milk:

1.   Soak the nuts overnight and drain them the next day.

2.   Blend the water and soaked nuts in a blender until a smooth consistency is attained.

3.   Add in the salt, vanilla extract, and maple syrup if you want and blend again until mixed well.

4.   Strain the mixture using a double layer of cheesecloth to isolate the pulp. Once done, add water to the milk to get your preferred consistency.

5.   Pour the nut milk into mason jars and store them if you want for up to 5 days.

6.   Cover the jars with lids and store in the refrigerator for up to 5 days.

Hemp Milk:

1.   Combine all the ingredients in a blender and blend for a few minutes or until a smooth consistency is attained.

2.   You can strain the excess seeds using a cheesecloth and store the hemp milk in mason jars for up to 5 days.

43 Gut Healing Bone Broth Latte

Servings: 2 | **Time:** 10 mins | **Difficulty**: Easy

Nutrients per serving: Calories: 161 kcal | Fat: 7.2g | Carbohydrates: 5.2g | Protein: 10.8g | Fiber: 0.9g

Ingredients

1 Tbsp. Coconut Oil

1/4 Tsp. Ginger, Ground

2 Cups Bone Broth

1/8 Tsp. Cayenne Pepper

1/8 Tsp. Turmeric Powder

1/8 Tsp. Black Pepper

1/8 Tsp. Sea Salt

Coconut Cream, To Taste (Optional)

Collagen Peptides (Optional)

Savory Latte Toppings (Optional)

Fresh Herbs

Green Onion, Chopped

Red Pepper Flakes

Method

1.   Pour bone broth into a saucepan and add all the ingredients in it except sea salt.

2.   Heat the mixture over medium flame while stirring constantly until combined.

3.   You can use an immersion blender to mix coconut cream if necessary.

4.   Blend well to make a frothy and creamy mixture.

5.   Pour into serving mugs and sprinkle seal salt on top.

6.   You can also use savory latte toppings for garnishing if you want.

44 Creamy Cocoa Coconut Low Carb Shake

Servings: 2 | **Time**: 5 mins | **Difficulty**: Easy

Nutrients per serving: Calories: 222 kcal | Fat: 23.1g | Carbohydrates: 5.4g | Protein: 2.5g | Fiber: 2.7g

Ingredients

2 Tbsps. Cocoa Powder

1/2 Tbsp. Almond Butter, Smooth

1 Cup Almond Or Coconut Milk, Unsweetened

2 Tbsps. Coconut MCT Oil

1/8 Tsp. Sea Salt

1/2 Cup Coconut Cream Additional Sweeteners (Optional)

Stevia Leaf Or Xylitol

Banana Or Maple Syrup Cinnamon

Berries

Method

1.   Combine all the ingredients in a blender and mix until a smooth consistency is attained.

2.   Add sweetener of your choice, if you want, and decant into the serving glasses and enjoy.

45 Low Carb Dark Chocolate Protein Smoothie

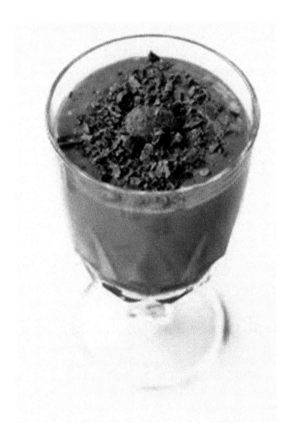

Servings: 1 | **Time**: 5 mins | **Difficulty:** Easy

Nutrients per serving: Calories: 220 kcal | Fat: 9g | Carbohydrates: 2.5g | Protein: 28.4g | Fiber: 19.5g

Ingredients

1 Cup Almond Milk, Unsweetened

1/4 Cup Avocado, Frozen

1/2 Tsp. Matcha Green Tea

2 Tbsps. Protein Powder, Zero Carb

1 Tbsp. Swerve Sweetener

1 Tbsp. Cocoa Powder, Dark

Method

1.   Combine all the ingredients in a blender and mix until a smooth consistency is attained.

2.   Decant into the serving glass and enjoy.

46 Mint Chocolate Green Smoothie

Servings: 2 | **Time**: 5 mins | **Difficulty**: Easy

Nutrients per serving: Calories: 359 kcal | Fat: 17.4g | Carbohydrates: 37.4g | Protein: 20.6g | Fiber: 10g

Ingredients

3/4 Cup Vanilla Almond Milk, Unsweetened

1/2 Cup Ice

1/2 Cup Kale, Packed Firmly

1/4 Cup Vanilla Protein Powder

1/4 Cup Vanilla Greek Yogurt (2%)

1/4 Cup Avocado, Mashed

1 Tbsp. Mini Chocolate Chips

1/4 Tsp. Peppermint Extract

1/2 Tbsp. Agave

Method

1.   Combine all the ingredients in a blender and mix until a smooth consistency is attained.

2.   Decant into the serving glasses and enjoy.

47 Low Carb Raspberry Cheesecake Shake

Servings: 1 | **Time:** 5 mins | **Difficulty**: Easy

Nutrients per serving: Calories: 560 kcal | Fat: 55g | Carbohydrates: 8g | Protein: 9g | Fiber: 3g

Ingredients

1/4 Cup Almond Milk, Unsweetened

1 Tsp. Butter, Unsalted (Cold)

1/4 Cup Heavy Cream

6-8 Raspberries, Fresh

1/4 Cup Cream Cheese

4 Tsps. Almond Flour

Ice (Optional)

Liquid Stevia, To Taste (Optional)

Method

1.   Put the almond milk, raspberries, heavy cream, and cream cheese in a vessel and blend using an immersion blender. Add the sweetener if you want. Transfer it into a serving glass.

2.   In a bowl, mix the almond flour and butter to form crumbs. Put these crumbs on top of the drink after adding ice, if you want, and serve.

48 Watermelon Smoothie

Servings: 1 | **Time:** 5 mins | **Difficulty**: Easy

Nutrients per serving: Calories: 39 kcal | Fat: 3g | Carbohydrates: 1g | Protein: 0g

Ingredients

3/4 Cup Lemon Lime Seltzer

1/8 Tsp. Xantham Gum

15 Drops Watermelon Flavoring Oil

8 Ice Cubes

1 Drop Vanilla Extract

2 Tbsps. Stevia

1 Drop Lemon Extract

1. Tbsp Heavy Cream

Method

1.   Combine all the ingredients in a blender and mix until a smooth consistency is attained.

2.   Decant into the serving glass and enjoy.

49   Low-Carb Blueberry Smoothie

Servings: 2 | **Time:** 5 mins | **Difficulty:** Easy

Nutrients per serving: Calories: 251 kcal | Fat: 22g | Carbohydrates: 6g | Protein: 8g | Fiber: 1g

Ingredients

1/4 Cup Cream Cheese

3/4 Cup Almond Milk, Unsweetened

1/2 Tsp. Vanilla Extract

1/2 Cup Ice

2 Tsps. Stevia/Erythritol Blend, Granulated

1/3 Cup Blueberries, Frozen

1-5 Drops Lemon Extract

1/4 Cup Heavy Whipping Cream

2 Tbsps. Collagen Peptides (Optional)

Method

1.   Combine all the ingredients in a blender and mix until a smooth consistency is attained.

2.   Decant into the serving glasses and enjoy.

50 Pumpkin Low Carb Smoothie With Salted Caramel

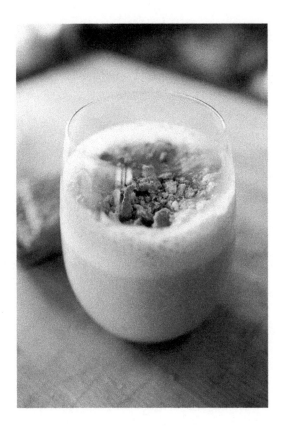

Servings: 1 | **Time:** 5 mins | **Difficulty:** Easy

Nutrients per serving: Calories: 245 kcal | Fat: 10.4g | Carbohydrates: 11.8g | Protein: 29g | Fiber: 6.4g

Ingredients

1 Cup Almond Milk

1/4 Avocado

2 Tbsps. Vanilla Protein Powder

1/4 Cup Pumpkin Puree

4 Ice Cubes

2 Tbsps. Caramel Syrup, Salted & Sugar-Free

Method

1.   Combine all the ingredients in a blender and mix until a smooth consistency is attained.

2.   Decant into the serving glass and enjoy.

Lightning Source UK Ltd.
Milton Keynes UK
UKHW020421070521
383233UK00001BA/30